Aortic Heart Valve Replacement: Through the Dark Curtain

By John Stibravy, Ph.D.

Edited by Tony Smith, Ph.D.

Table of Contents

Preface

Wild Thing, You Make My Heart Sing

– The Troggs (1966)

IF YOU:

Can't sleep at night lying flat without discomfort…

Can't catch your breath after going up stairs…

Can't get up the stairs without stopping…

Can't carry packages without being very tired…

Experience chest pain during exercise…

Pant when walking on level ground…

Can only sleep on one side…

Lose weight for no reason…

Have a heart rate that seems fast and irregular…

Suffer a pounding heart when at rest, especially upon waking up…

Then you may be headed towards the operating table and a procedure known as aortic heart valve replacement. This book is for you.

Introduction: Fear and Shock

Everyone who goes through heart valve replacement surgery is never going to forget that day in the cardiologist's office when, after the test results are in, the doctor, while holding the patient's charts and papers and smiling reassuringly, tells the patient what is wrong: a bad heart valve. Eventually, the doctor will arrive at the bottom line: the patient needs open heart surgery to replace a heart valve. That means having one's chest cut open, the heart stopped, being hooked to a heart-lung machine while the bad valve is cut out and a replacement sewn in, the heart restarted, being taking off the machine, and sewn up to recover. No wonder a person is scared! One has every right to be frightened about having the heart stopped and a piece cut out and replaced. Everyone is *terrified*.

One day when I was at the cardiology office, one of the nurse practitioners was running an EKG on me after we had set the date for the operation, and she asked if I were scared. I said I was terrified. Her reply was, "Good, at least you're honest. I'll see you after the operation." She *did*, too. So be honest with yourself and your loved ones and friends. Unless your faith is a supreme part of your life, you are going to be terrified when you leave the doctor's office after receiving the news. I didn't tell anyone for days what was wrong with me, because the news was so shocking.

Overview

If you *do* need to have a heart valve replaced, the procedure is straightforward. The only cure for a bad heart valve is surgery, and the only currently reliable surgery is open heart. While there are other procedures that are less invasive now undergoing testing, they were not the most effective life-saving techniques back in 2009, when I underwent surgery. Based on additional research conducted in May 2022, it would seem not a lot has changed in the years that have passed. Today, as was the case back then, medicine can perhaps control the symptoms for a while – maybe *years* – but drugs are not a cure and people generally become worse. It's best to do the operation before the patient's decline becomes too severe.

In simple terms, the surgical team is going to open the patient's sternum, stop the heart using a cold solution, and hook up the patient to a heart-lung machine that will circulate the blood and breathe for the patient. The team will then cut out the bad heart valve and replace the valve with either a tissue or artificial valve, restart the heart, while at the same time leaving the patient for a while on a breathing machine, then sew up the chest incision. If all goes well, the patient recovers in four to eight weeks depending on age, medical health, and type of job the patient will return to. Back to work in four weeks is a *rapid* recovery. Patients usually need six to eight weeks for recovery.

Chapter 1: How it Started (August – December 2008)

There are lots of ways of identifying a heart valve going bad. For me, the trouble started in early August in the heat of summer. When it was very hot, I panted when I was just walking around outdoors. I panted walking from the car into the school building. I panted going up the stairs. I panted at athletics, but only if it were very hot, above 90 degrees. If the temperatures were more moderate outdoors, I didn't pant at all. I told myself it was just the heat. But by the end of August the pattern kept going. On hot days I panted. On mild days I didn't.

I started losing weight, too, and people began to notice. I ate more, and *still* lost weight. From November to March I lost 30 pounds without trying to lose anything. Weight just seemed to vanish away. I kept getting thinner and thinner.

In August, I went to see my general practitioner for my annual visit for blood pressure and cholesterol prescription renewals. I almost never became sick, and rarely had to go see her. While I was there, I mentioned that I was panting a lot and couldn't seem to get enough oxygen on hot days. She ran an EKG, said I was developing a heart murmur, and referred me to a cardiologist nearby for a consultation and evaluation a week later. Her comment when she called the cardiologist was that I should be seen sooner rather than later, and this consultation should not be postponed. Clearly, she knew more than she was willing to say this early. That reticence was alarming, but I didn't ask for details.

A week later, I went to see the cardiologist. Well-known, well-respected, board certified and chairman of the county cardiology association, and all that. He listened with his stethoscope. Yes, I had a heart murmur. Time for testing. The tests were scheduled for two weeks later.

If one believes only unhealthy people head towards the operating room at a young age, one must rethink one's beliefs. I was only 59 when the trouble started, a non-smoker, an athletic coach in good shape, and very active. I went up and down the stairs 20 times a day at my school. I taught 18- to 22-year-olds with two hours of athletics, four days a week. I rowed boats and did lots of outdoor work such as cutting wood.

I had longevity genes on my father's side, with my father living past 94 and his mother living to see 103. There was lots of heart trouble on my *mother's* side of the family, but nothing at an early age. There was never any heart valve trouble among my parents. My parents' and grandparents' heart trouble was all on my mother's side. Both grandparents died of heart failure, but they were in their 80s. So there was no reason to suspect any early trouble ahead. I split firewood every week, rowed two days a week, shoveled gravel for community service projects, and worked outdoors a lot. I led an *active* life.

The initial tests were scheduled in two weeks, right across the street from the cardiologist's office. Testing day was the usual putting of IV leads in the veins, then waiting a while. In fact, after the prep was done, I went home and watched TV for two hours, then drove back to the testing center. I lay on a table while a camera rotated around, 360 degrees, taking heart pictures. After that, it was on to the treadmill test.

Most people are probably familiar with the treadmill test. A patient is hooked up to bunches of heart and chest leads, then one walks while the treadmill tilts upwards, placing an increasing load on the heart. I had no trouble with the treadmill test and showed no symptoms. No chest pain, and because it was air conditioned in the treadmill room, I didn't pant much, either.

When one has only a minute of walking left in one's legs, one tells the doctor, and one is injected with a radioactive dye. Then, one goes back to the camera table and more photos are taken of where the heart is sending that dye. For me, much of the dye was going in the wrong direction through the aortic valve. In simple terms, the valve was leaking blood backwards, even though I had no symptoms at all on the treadmill. The doctor recommended surgery soon. I said, "Let's see what medicine will do first." Sometimes medicine can control the symptoms and postpone surgery, sometimes for years. Sometimes it doesn't.

The weather cooled down. I was on heart medications, and all symptoms went away. There were no symptoms in September and

October. I thought everything was going to be okay. In November, I was in New York State when the temperature dropped to 20 degrees.

Walking indoors to an athletic event, I started to pant, and carrying gear up two flights of stairs nearly finished me off. I panted all the way up the steps, and couldn't walk when I reached the top. I leaned against the wall, panting, unable to walk along the hallway. I simply couldn't breathe, couldn't get over the cold air and the exertion of the steps. It took five minutes before I could walk down the hallway. The rest of the day I used the elevator. There were no more symptoms the rest of the trip, but once was scary enough. I tried to avoid stairs after this incident.

My first cardiologist, working alone, was exceptionally booked with patients, so I made an appointment to switch cardiologists in December to a large cardiology group. Unfortunately, the appointment had to be canceled due to an emergency on the group's end, and rescheduled for January. The holidays came and went, and no symptoms were present. I stayed on medication.

In January, I had to cancel the appointment with the new cardiologist due to an ice storm; still, there were no serious symptoms except that on very cold days, I panted. I shoveled snow and panted, but there was no chest pain, and no other symptoms at all. There was no discomfort when shoveling snow, either. I hoped things would stabilize and I could avoid the surgery.

Chapter 2: Emergency Room Trip (February 2009)

By February, not only did the weight loss continue, but now my face looked like something from Halloween: all bone. My color went bad, too, and in a hurry. A pale, white, pasty, washed-out look took over by February. People noticed *that*, too. I did not look hearty and robust any longer. Thin, bad color, barely able to walk up one flight of steps without stopping – that was becoming my life. I was spending 10 hours in bed each night and waking up still tired. It got to the point that on every flight of steps, I had to stop and pant awhile. I tried to always use elevators.

On February 15, I had a bad day. I panted all day, felt dizzy, and had heart palpitations and irregular heartbeats. I spent the afternoon coaching my team while leaning up against the wall, unable to stand without support. It turned out I was having a bad reaction to one of the heart drugs. Irregular heartbeats came and went. After dinner, I went to a walk-in clinic and had an EKG done.

The doctor, who looked about 18 and still seemed to be in high school, said that the waves were upside down and recommended going to the Emergency Room. I asked if this visit could be postponed until the following day so I could sleep in my own bed that night. He thought that was unwise, so I went home and packed a bag, and at 11 p.m., I was off to the Emergency Room.

In triage, I waited two hours before being taken in due to a high load of accident cases coming in. I was then hooked up to a heart monitor, placed in a cubicle, and after seeing assorted doctors and being awake all night, was admitted at 6 a.m. the next morning and went to my real room for evaluation, where I finally met one of the young doctors from my new cardiology group. The nurses were wonderfully competent. The most difficult part of being in a hospital bed was trying not to worry about what was happening at my job while I was in the hospital. The symptoms, naturally, had ceased. I just as well could have gone home and gone to bed the night before.

The doctor from my cardio group came in for a detailed recent history and evaluation, and I was kept for observation. I told him about the series of canceled appointments and that there were generally no symptoms except some panting, until this week. He was concerned. I remember him saying, "This is your heart, not something unimportant."

I had a beautiful room, great nurses, and spent the day reading the Bible, enjoying the fine view, and doing nothing. Sitting around was a vast difference from the high-pressure job I worked at the time. People have suggested that all of this heart trouble was caused by working a high-pressure job, but the truth is that the causes of most heart trouble can be so varied from one individual to the next that the cause of a specific person's heart trouble may never be really known.

Various patient services people came by. The people from the chaplain's office came by. All the while, I waited. The doctors ordered another echocardiogram for the next morning at 11 a.m. There was a long line of patients waiting for echocardiograms, so it was 2 p.m. before I went down for the testing. The results were *not* good. My EF

("Ejection Factor," a measure of the heart's efficiency, with 70 or better being the norm) was dropping slowly, and the valve was no better. My hope that this could be controlled by medicine was fading. The doctors wanted a heart cath done while I was at the hospital.

In the meantime, I read, ate the fine hospital food which really was good, and rested – trying not to think about my job getting out of control while I was away. Just as the line for an echo was long, so was the line for a heart cath. It was going to be a few days before I could get the heart cath done since I wasn't critical yet, but the doctors thought it best to keep me around for observation and more tests.

I'd been admitted on a Monday, but on Wednesday, while I was quietly reading and taking in the fine view, people suddenly decided I was wasting a needed bed. So, I went home and back to work. The heart cath was scheduled for 10 a.m. the following Monday, a week after I had been admitted through the ER.

Chapter 3: The Heart Cath (February 2009)

The heart cath procedure seems scary because one signs a lot of waiver forms, but as long as there are thoracic surgeons in the hospital where the cath is being done, there's little to fear. There is a chance of the wire used in the procedure puncturing a vein, but it's very rare. The greatest danger may be falling off the narrow table. One feels as if one is going to fall off, but it doesn't happen. Patients check in early, usually around 6 to 7 a.m., and go through the usual procedure of getting into the hospital gown, having two IV leads inserted in the same arm because both may be used during the procedure to administer drugs, signing forms, and waiting. There's a good deal of waiting.

Next, one is transported to a holding area just outside the procedure room for a little more paperwork, then into the procedure room, which is mostly a narrow table and a bunch of monitors. One's groin area is shaved, and a nurse administers a sedative which keeps the patient barely awake. One can talk and respond if questioned, but otherwise one has no sense of time. There's no pain where a small incision is made in the groin at a vein, through which a thin wire is moved to the heart for a look-around. The heart is examined to see if any bypass work will be needed when the valve is replaced, and the valve is photographed so that the proper valve size can be preselected. In general, this is a chance to see if more work than just valve replacement is needed (such as a bypass) by examining the heart, taking photos, and monitoring everything.

Sometimes the patient can watch too, but you may not wish to do so. You're right on the edge of sleeping, but not quite. Frankly, it's very easy. When the cardiologist is finished, the patient is stitched and bandaged on the inside of the thigh where the wire has been inserted, and the area will probably turn black and blue. One should *not* pull those stitches loose.

Afterwards, patients are moved to a recovery room for a nap and a sandwich. Patients must stay on their backs for three to four hours of watching TV and sleeping, then go home if one is just in for an outpatient procedure. Overall, it's a very easy day with nothing to fear. The doctor will come by and tell the patient the results of the heart cath.

My doctors wanted to get right inside my heart and operate. In a polite way, they weren't so optimistic. I asked for time to finalize everything. Will, power of attorney, living will, organ donor card, safe deposit box signatures…all the things that the legal people said should be done. I also thought it very important to be in the right frame of mind and at peace before undergoing the operation.

The doctors and I looked at the calendar, and we agreed I could have 16 days. I picked March 4th for the operation. They weren't happy about the wait, but I argued that a content patient would recover faster than a rushed and anxious one.

After the heart cath, I went home and went back to teaching.

Chapter 4: Sixteen Critical Days to Prepare

The doctors changed some of the meds and increased the dosages as a stop-gap measure. I felt a little better, but it was clear that the days' activities were going to be limited now. I could no longer teach standing up; I sat through classes now. I panted walking down the hallway to class from my office. It seemed like a long walk from my office to the classroom. Some nights were *bad*…I was dizzy, unable to lie flat without discomfort, and unable to sleep more than a few seconds at a time. I slept sitting up, so as not to be dizzy and disoriented.

It was remarkable how the decline accelerated after my February ER visit. The meds were changed again, and some of the symptoms improved. Coaching athletics meant leaning against a wall now all the time or sitting in a chair, trying to just get through it. I could barely walk from the athletic area back to my car. Most of the day, I just sat.

One of the cardiologists had said in August that I eventually wouldn't be able to get across the room. I didn't believe it in August. By March, I *believed* him. My ability to walk up one flight of steps was borderline. When I arrived at the top of a set of steps, I panted. I panted at *any* exertion now. It was as if I couldn't get enough oxygen ever, and my EF was about 40 percent. Not all that low – except when compared to a *healthy* person, who would function at 70 percent or better. It became all I could do to walk anywhere at all. All the time now, I had to stop halfway up a flight of steps. Sometimes I couldn't even make it halfway before stopping. It was three steps and wait. Then another three steps.

My general practitioner had recommended doing the operation at 30 percent EF. The cardiologists said, "No way." It would be at 40 percent or not at all, meaning I would cease to exist by fall at the latest. Once the EF fell under a certain point, the operation couldn't be done because I wouldn't survive it.

In addition to the legal paperwork that a patient should prepare, one should also consider what *not* to leave behind for the kids to find in case the patient doesn't survive. I spent days throwing away photos, letters, souvenirs, mementoes…stuff I didn't want my son to find. Some items in one's life really are personal, and at a watershed event such as this operation, it's best to junk a lot of stuff rather than have it found. It usually only means something to the patient anyway, a longing for the better past when life seemed to stretch out forever into a distant future that suddenly has a termination date waiting out there. So, bite the bullet and throw away the past. One really doesn't want one's kids reading love letters from 40 years ago, or seeing photos of people whom the child will never meet or even be able to find. Let it all go into the trash. An operation such as this really does divide the past from the present, so throw things away and go out to a big dinner and forget all the people from your past. They are gone. You hope *not* to be.

Have a thorough housecleaning not only of stuff, but of *people*. If there are people in one's life causing stress, or unresolved issues haunting a person, maybe this is the time to resolve those issues so that, on the day of the operation, one can focus one's mind on survival and not be thinking about unresolved issues that should've been dealt with. People pass on eventually, but one's survival after this operation may be enhanced by a proper frame of mind and a positive viewpoint. So, go deal with people and *resolve* things.

Do not go gentle into that good night

Old age should burn and rave at close of day

Rage, rage, against the dying of the light.

– Dylan Thomas (1914 - 1953)

Chapter 5: Some Advice for Dealing With the Operation

If one remembers nothing from this book except the following, then this book was worth studying.

Tip #1: It Is Better Not to Know Too Much About This Operation

A person I knew who had this operation done wanted to know nothing at all. He let his son know everything instead. I think that old fellow was right. Don't know *too much*. If you have kids, let the kids know all they want to. Maybe they'll be nicer to you. If your spouse is elderly, maybe your spouse shouldn't know too much either, as knowing things may upset your spouse (and you, as well). One doesn't need to be upset when facing this operation.

A patient can watch videos of the procedure online, obtain medical texts, and see pictures of what will be done. I strongly advise you *not* to do this. Talk in general terms with the surgeon. Ignorance is bliss. Don't upset yourself and everyone around you more than you'll be already. Believe me, you do *not* want to watch an online video of this operation, nor do you want to see color pictures of the surgical steps. *Don't do it.* Go have some wine instead. Go to a party. Don't prowl the internet looking for information. Remember the story of Pandora's Box? *Don't open it.*

In particular, do not think about or ask about the heart-lung machine. While you are asleep, a machine will breathe and circulate blood for you. Essentially, it will be your heart while yours is stopped. The technicians running this machine are critical to your life, and you *should* inquire about their expertise so you'll be reassured. No surgeon is going to tell you that these people are all new and just learning. Instead, the surgeon will give you comforting words about the team members. Complications can arise, but they are rare, so don't ask. It's just more to think about.

The machine is hooked into your veins to circulate your blood with tubes going over to the machine, so don't think about *that*, either. You won't know anything about what is going on – and you don't *want* to know beforehand.

I had asked the first cardiologist what if I didn't survive the operation. His answer was, "Then you don't wake up." That was *not* the positive answer I'd hoped for. I guess he was tired of people asking the same question. So, there's something *else* not to think about. You simply won't ever wake up if you don't survive the operation. Go have some wine and don't think about this. Maybe have *lots* of wine.

Tip #2: How You Recover Is Very Much an Individual Response

Some people can't sleep lying down after they go home, but would rather sleep in a chair. I slept lying down all right, but only on the left side or on my back. For months, it was uncomfortable sleeping on my right side. No specific reason, I was just uncomfortable. Today, it's the other way. Sleeping on the *left* side is uncomfortable. Whatever. Your results will be *your* results.

I read all over the internet about how people don't do better after this operation, and some seem to be worse. *Ignore this.* You are *you*. A positive attitude is everything, and no one else's results are of much use to you. Ignore these anecdotes and predictions of how long you'll need to recover. I strongly advise *not* reading everyone's blogs about this operation. Ignore them.

The first cardiologist said four to eight weeks off from work. My reply was, "No way." When I had my appendix removed, I was back at work in a week. I thought I could be back in a month this time, not sitting home for eight weeks. In reality, I was back to work in my office four weeks after the operation, or three weeks after going home. You control your recovery. Recovery does not control you.

Tip #3: Find a Team Which Only Does These Types of Operations

Everyone on the team should be doing lots of valve replacements. You don't want a team which rotates people through different specialties. Your team should be a dedicated team whose members work together all the time. That means *everyone*: nurses, doctors, anesthesiologists, phlebotomists – *everyone* – with someone in charge whom you trust (usually the head surgeon). You want a dedicated heart team at a hospital that has a good patient survival rate, and you can often find survival rates listed online.

The average immediate mortality rate for this operation is five percent. The long-term survival rate is 60 percent at 10 years, but there is a wide variation in the underlying health of people who survive the operation but have other problems. So, ignore these statistics, too. You are *you* – not a pile of statistics. Statistics make one worry, so ignore them.

Tip #4: Do Some *Research!*

Investigate the hospital and surgeon online and via public records available. Check survival rates for the hospital where the operation will be done. *Ask around.* There's lots of information available online, but by asking around, you might discover patients who used your surgeon, maybe years ago, and survived. It's reassuring while you're at the oil change place to find the fellow sitting next to you has survived the same operation from years ago, with the same surgeon you have. So, tell people what you're facing. You may be surprised whom you meet.

In general, research seems to show that the more of these operations a hospital does, the better the survival rate. The same is true for the surgeon. There seems to be no difference in survival rates for time of day or day of the week, with *one exception*: Survival rates for a *Friday afternoon operation* seem worse than any other day of the week.

The best option appears to be an experienced surgeon with a set team, dedicated cardiac ICU, and dedicated cardiac hospital floor with experienced nurses, and an operation time not on a Friday afternoon, in a hospital where lots of these operations are done. The heart cath should be done at a hospital with thoracic surgeons available. Large cardiology groups with numerous doctors and nurse practitioners seem somewhat better than a lone cardiologist, if only because there are more people readily available to help the patient and consult with each other, should complications arise.

The care team of the surgeons, cardiology group, social workers, nurses, dieticians, physical therapists, chaplain's assistants, counselors, and many other professionals is very important to one's recovery. Pick the cardiologist and surgeon with some thought. If, when you meet the surgeon to discuss the operation, you don't feel comfortable, then it's time to find another surgeon. The same is true for the cardiologist. Don't be shy about changing to a different doctor early in the development of your case – while there's still time -- if you don't seem compatible with the doctor. Your relationship with them is sort of like a marriage, and if you know it won't work, then express your concerns.

I might not have done the operation except that I was so comfortable with the surgeon, who had been recommended by my original cardiologist, that I felt a strong sense of trust and a certainty that everything would go well after talking to him. One of the things I liked best was a sense that I could ask whatever I wanted, and he took plenty of time to discuss the operation. In fact, I was the one who ended our discussion. I never felt that he had to run off somewhere. We only met once, but it was enough to know he was good at his profession. With that in mind, find people you trust and listen to your own reactions to the doctors. Don't stay with someone you're not comfortable with.

Tip #5: Get Your Mental Frame of Mind Together

There's more about this topic later, but meditation before the operation, prayer, reading religious texts…anything along this line is useful. Quiet reflection somewhere, whether in a religious building, or out in a nature setting, or in a tanning booth, or lying drunk on the lawn, staring up at the moon, is useful. Meditation – whatever one's religion – seems to encourage a positive mental frame of mind and better odds of a rapid recovery.

Make final arrangements, get the legal items in order, and tell people what you want done if you don't survive. This operation isn't like getting a broken bone set. This is going to be betting your life when you're on the operating table. Accept that and prepare well. Listen to music, watch funny movies, and get things in order so that, on the morning of the operation, you're at peace. Prepare *well*. This is the ultimate bet of one's life. Make the odds favor your survival.

Chapter 6: Preop Day

We had a blizzard again. I was the only one on the highway to the hospital for the preop workup. This workup is not a big deal. Patients have some briefings, sign more forms, and give blood and urine for testing. I was the only person to show up for a morning preop appointment due to the snow, and I was done in two hours.

I went over to look at the multimillion-dollar gym and treadmill facility for heart patients who are recovering. It's staffed with trainers and nurses, and people on treadmills are wearing heart monitors. Everyone was very friendly and said hello. "We'll be seeing you in a few weeks," they said. The patients explained the reassuring feeling of having a nurse right there for this rehab work, and of being in a hospital when doing their daily running.

It struck me that a lot of patients were afraid to go *live*, and now spent their days hanging around the hospital after they'd run, just waiting for an incident to fell them like a cut-down tree. It would indeed be handy to have the nurses right there, close by. They could save one's life in the event of a heart attack, and are a fine emotional crutch. I decided I would *not* be exercising at the hospital. I had the distinct feeling that many of these people were afraid to go far from the hospital, whether they were in the running room, cafeteria, or newspaper shop.

Most hospitals have cardiac support group meetings so survivors of heart events can encourage each other. I'm sorry, but being in a group of people with the same sort of heart problems just isn't my cup of tea. I planned to surround myself with 19- to 22-year-olds who are healthy and look great. I want to be around people who are beautiful and handsome. Being with the young keeps one young. I've always had the feeling that being surrounded by ill people is a good way to feel ill. Thus, think carefully before getting into one of these support groups, as it may make you feel old. I never went to the exercise center and never went to a group meeting. Instead, I picked up an epee and fenced against 19-year-olds. I *lost* a lot, but I felt great when I would nail one of them right between the eyes. So, choose your surroundings and the people around you with care after the operation. Don't make yourself old.

Chapter 7: Changing One's Mind About the Operation

People may be tempted to call the whole operation off, especially if they feel better after lots of rest. One may have some good days suddenly, and it seems as if everything is okay. There may be a great desire just to go home the morning of the operation and refuse to do it. If one does this without a medical reason after everything is set to go, then several things are apt to happen. Your surgeon and cardiologist may politely tell you to go find other doctors, the hospital may be unwilling to schedule another operation date, you may have to pay for everyone's time, and you are not really better at all and will continue to decline until you will be too weak to have the operation.

I'll put this directly to you: If your EF is continuing to drop and the symptoms increase, you either have the operation or you're going to die relatively soon, probably within months. Once your EF drops below 20 percent, you won't be able to walk to the dining room table, nor will you want to. Decision time is when the EF is at 40 - 55 percent, based on your health and your cardiologist's and surgeon's recommendations. If the EF is at 20 percent, no one is going to risk doing an operation on you, as you won't survive it. You'll just make the hospital's numbers look bad. Feeling good is an illusion, and one that can prove fatal.

Yes, you can change your mind and stop the operation, maybe enter Hospice, or go home and just be dead in a few months. Drugs are not a cure, and the experimental minimally invasive and experimental insertion of a new valve into a vein may come with a high mortality rate. The mortality rate may eventually improve for new types of procedures, but for now, if drugs don't control the symptoms well, then it's this operation or stay home to die. Those are the simple facts.

If your cardiologist says you need the operation, then go do it. It's your chance for *life*. Years ago, there was no such option. If you are well enough to have the operation, then you now have the choice to *live*. Your great-grandparents didn't have this option. They died from a bad valve.

The winter after I had the operation, I was shoveling snow, and the fellow shoveling out his car next to mine told me about his grandfather, who died of a bad valve. He was just 41 years old and died in the 1930s. A valve replacement operation didn't exist back then. You, however, are lucky. You have a *chance*.

Chapter 8: The Operation (March 4, 2009)

Well, the day has arrived. Try to be cheery about this day so you don't depress the entire family. At least let them remember you as optimistic and upbeat about life, even if you're not.

Patients have to shower with antiseptic soap twice, sleep on newly-cleaned sheets the last night at home, and sleep in clean pajamas to reduce the risk of infection. Infection after a heart operation can be serious and rapidly fatal, so it's best to try to avoid this. Lots of things after the operation can be serious, so one should do as told to make recovery the best experience possible.

The patient will be told when to appear at the hospital and what to bring, such as legal documents and other paperwork. Family can accompany a patient through the preliminary procedures such as checking in and getting into the hospital gown with the open rear. Don't bother being modest. You'll be on a table soon, fully exposed anyway. Nurses know all about the human anatomy, so don't be too concerned about what they're going to see. They've seen *everything*. Bring warm socks, as it's always cold in hospitals, and ask for some blankets.

Again, the nurse is going to set up the IVs into your veins that the anesthesiologist will use. You'll probably be given some sort of relaxing medication in the form of a shot, and the lights will be dimmed somewhat. A same-gender nurse is going to come shave all the hair off your chest (males) and groin using an electric shaver (you don't want hair in the incision site). For some parts of this procedure the patient will lie down, and for other parts, the patient will stand up. It's a little weird standing naked and talking with the nurse while having one's hair shaved off, but it has to be done for the patient's own good. Again, get over trying to be modest. Nurses have seen hundreds of patients just like you. The sheets on the patient's bed will be changed afterwards before the patient lies down again.

It's time to say goodbye to friends and family. This goodbye should be brief, so as not to start anyone crying. "I love you and I'll see you in a few hours" is sufficient. Kids should generally be said goodbye to at home, in a comfortable environment, then left with a family member overnight on the night before the operation. Advice to the kids about life, marriage, and school should be given at home, *not* at the hospital. Let them remember you in your favorite chair, maybe reading a story to them or playing a video game – not in a hospital prep area. It will terrify the child (children) and make you feel bad when they leave. The long goodbyes and reminisces should be done at home, days before. Family members will see you in four to five hours, but you will not see them until the next day.

A professional family support group of some sort can be very useful at this time, and should be pre-arranged. All hospitals have a chaplain's office or spiritual office, and prior arrangements can be made to have a chaplain or religious person meet the family members and stay with them while the patient undergoes the operation, perhaps staying at the chapel or other meditation room rather than the cafeteria.

The chaplain's office is typically well-prepared for these operations, and very competent regardless of the patient's outcome or the family's religion. The counselor assigned may not be of the family's specific religion, but they're accustomed to working and supporting all religious needs and views. Contact the hospital chaplain's office and request that a counselor meet the family when you arrive on operation day, at the check-in area. The chaplain's office people are used to meeting families and have access to all the admission areas and wards. They'll meet you and your family at the check-in location, and have probably already checked your check-in time and operation time on the schedule before you arrive (provided you contacted them a few days before).

There are places available in the hospital for the family to pray or meditate, and lots of counselors available. In fact, from now on, the operation is more difficult for the *family* than it is for the patient. The family, after all, will be thinking and probably worrying. The patient, however, *won't* be. They'll be asleep, and will know nothing.

I tried to implant into my head one thought to be there when I woke up. All that morning of the operation, I said to myself that the first thing I would think when I woke up is: "I *survived*." I said this to myself, over and over. It *worked*. It really *was* the very first thing I thought the next day, when I dimly saw the wall in front of me and the railing of the bed. Implanting an idea into one's mind before the operation, something simple, may very well work. One fellow I heard about asked a nurse to tell him over and over while he was asleep that he was *loved*. It may have worked: he had a fast recovery from the operation. Thus, implanting an idea – something simple – into your mind before you're put to sleep might well be worth it.

You'll be moved to a waiting area close to the operating room. Here, in your relaxed state, you'll meet the anesthesiologist. No doubt the anesthesiologist will be jolly and upbeat, and will cheer you up a lot. Anesthesiologists are always like that. I've never met an anesthesiologist who'd tell a patient that the experience coming up was going to be awful. It never happens. These doctors must study being cheerful in medical school, because they always seem jolly when putting patients to sleep.

The room is likely to be dim, and if you tell the anesthesiologist you're very nervous and that the relaxing shot you had downstairs did nothing at all to help you relax, they're likely to say something like, "I have something more effective." And they *do*. In fact, that comment is probably the last comment you'll hear from them. You may feel a needle, and that's it. You'll then be asleep. I told the anesthesiologist that the shot downstairs had no effect at all, and that I knew perfectly well what was going on around me, and could see and hear everything. He picked up a syringe, stuck it in me, and that was the last thing I said for about 20 hours. I must've been out in two seconds after that injection.

People have asked me if, when my heart was stopped, there were angels or heaven or lights or anything. Sorry, but the answer is there was nothing. Modern anesthesia, if you've never had it before, is *nothing* like sleeping. It's not even like the anesthesia of the 1950s. When one sleeps, one normally dreams and tosses about and has an awareness of what is going on and that one is in bed. Under today's anesthesia, there is nothing at all. No awareness, no time. One's blood moves and one

breathes via a heart-lung machine while the heart is stopped, but there's

no awareness of time. Whether one is out for two, six, or 12 hours,

there's no sense of time passing. There is nothing, and one doesn't

notice there's nothing.

You're alive and don't know it. In some ways, this is the most

unsettling part of the operation. There exists no sense at all of what is

being done inside you. It's best to try not think about this aspect of the

operation, or you may get yourself riled up and worried. If you *do* start

thinking about this, go have some wine until these thoughts go away. If

you can't sleep *after* the operation due to these thoughts, tell the doctor

and get a pill. Don't be brave. Be scared and take a pill and go to sleep at

night. Otherwise, one gets into a complete derailing frenzy and *never*

sleeps. Go to sleep and *heal*. If a pill is what it takes to sleep, then take

the pill.

The people who went to the hospital with me asked the doctors

around noon how things were going. My operation was to start at 10 a.m., but due to an emergency, the team put me in a corner while I slept, and the operation began at 12:30. When asked how I was doing, the doctors said they hadn't started, and that I was asleep in the corner. Everyone laughed at the picture of me sleeping in a corner somewhere. That's probably not a joke. I probably really *was* asleep in some corner of the hospital. Perhaps there are corners whose only purpose is to house sleeping patients waiting for their operation.

There will be no sense at all to you of how long you're asleep. The family will fidget. You will *not*. You will know nothing.

What would you like to do after you recover? Make a list!

Chapter 9: Wake Up!

You hope to wake up in the cardiac ICU sometime. If you don't, you'll never know it, and your next stop is the funeral home – but it's best not to think about *that*, either. There are *lots* of things you shouldn't think about. You will have an R.N. assigned to you, often one R.N. to one patient, with a doctor nearby. Within *seconds* of your bed. Within *feet* of you. Some of these ICUs are set up in a circle so the doctor can see into each room. A central desk monitors each patient, and you'll be wearing a heart monitor that sends signals to the central monitoring desk. You'll be very well cared for.

You'll wake up in a sort of not quite conscious state, like being in a dream but more fragmented. You'll be drugged and generally immobile. A tube may be down your throat, attached to a machine to help you breathe. You may wish to discuss this with your doctor beforehand, because waking up to a tube in your throat may be unsettling, to say the least. There may be some difficult decisions about having a machine to help you breathe, relative to your age, when you wake up. Keep in mind that everyone on the medical staff wants you off that machine soon, just as you do. If you can't breathe on your own, the machine does it for you until you can. You'll like being put *back* on the machine even less than being on it in the first place, so try to relax if you're on one for a while.

The operation was about three to four hours, with my heart stopped about an hour. For me, while waking up, I have a dim fragment of memory of fighting off people with my left arm, flailing around violently, then nothing. I think the doctors put me back to sleep. I'd told the doctor that if I woke up and there was a breathing tube down my throat, I'd instinctively try to rip it out. I think that's what happened.

The next thing I knew, it was morning and the sun was shining into my ICU room. There was no breathing tube. I was breathing on my own, and I felt as if I had a good night's sleep. The nurse gave me a cloth bath to wipe off the yellow disinfectant markings. The patient's body is coated in yellow to indicate the patient has been disinfected, and a nurse will eventually wash off that coloring. Next, two very strong nursing assistants are going to get the patient sitting up. Then, with the patient's arms around their necks, they'll move the patient a few feet into a chair. The patient will totally rely on their help, and will have no energy to move or do anything. I was 180 pounds and an athletic coach, yet I couldn't take a single step without the two of them holding me up.

The patient will sit in a chair and have no energy to move at all. Two electric leads will be hanging out of the chest in case the patient needs a pacemaker suddenly. A urinary catheter will be in with a urine bag somewhere, there will be multiple IV or syringe leads stitched into a vein in the neck in case the patient needs a sudden IV, and there will be a drain tube coming out the bottom of the stomach to drain fluids away from the heart and chest. Surprisingly, none of these things will bother the patient at all. The survivor of the operation really won't care about these minor things.

One sits in a chair and one's family and friends will come to bring cheer. You'll have no energy at all to deal with being cheered up, and a brief visit will seem like an endurance run. Brief visits are best. It's important to sit up to prevent pneumonia and other lung troubles, so the patient sits up in the ICU room. Various people (staff, family, etc.) will visit the patient, and the patient will look at them, and nothing much will bother the patient, who feels lucky to be awake and alive, and really doesn't want a lot of visitors and commotion.

I strongly advise *not* allowing children to see you in ICU. Wait until you have your wits together to deal with children. They may not be allowed in the cardiac ICU to begin with. Children certainly should not see the patient unconscious in ICU before waking up. It's not such a nice sight, especially if the patient is on a breathing machine, so leave the kids at home. They are better off there for a few days, and you don't want them remembering you this way. Other than not having much physical energy, the patient will feel pretty good, and there will be no pain.

Someone will bring the patient something to drink (maybe juice). I tried apple. Five minutes after I drank it, the nurse was away checking something, and I started throwing up violently. The housekeeping person scrubbing the floor ran out for the nurse who came right in, plugged a syringe into the neck leads, shot the injection into me, and my nausea was gone in a matter of seconds. It worked that quickly. I had some more apple juice.

After 30 minutes of the patient enduring sitting up, and visitors being chatty when one doesn't feel like chatting, the two nursing assistants will put the patient back into bed. A patient should expect to be as weak as can be when first woken up, but one may regain their strength in a hurry. If there are no complications, the patient is moved to a cardiac floor into a regular room with a roommate, where they'll stay for five to seven days.

One has made the first step toward a successful recovery upon leaving the ICU. Leaving the ICU soon is a good step towards going home, and a good sign of future recovery. You don't leave ICU if you're not doing okay.

Chapter 10: Recovery

Your recovery time is yours and no one else's. Above all else, what everyone has said about their experience after the operation has little relevance to you as an individual. The hospital stay is typically five to seven days. It could be longer but is rarely shorter. If you're thinking you can go home in three days, forget it.

The cardiac nursing staff is usually very experienced, often with over 20 years of nursing time per person. I found that, in the hospital I was in, everyone was good at their job, from food service to housekeeping, to the CNAs to the R.N.s, to the doctors. Maybe this was a superb hospital, but I was very impressed. Everyone felt as if they were part of the recovery team – and they definitely were.

Each patient is given some sort of cloth heart pillow to hug. It'll hurt to cough, and you should try your best not to sneeze. Where the sternum has been put back together is going to hurt if one coughs. This is another good reason not to get any sort of infection that will cause coughing. When one leaves the hospital, they should carry the pillow along to all doctors' appointments. Coughing and sneezing is going to hurt for at least a month. Hug the pillow tightly to the sternum and the pain will be lessened considerably.

The remaining hospital stay is composed mostly of doing nothing except reading or watching TV, eating, and resting. Each patient has a wireless heart monitor on all the time, but it's small and won't be a bother. Patients will take a lot of pills, have some IVs, be on blood thinners, be checked every couple of hours all night long, and generally be watched over. After the first day, patients will be encouraged to get out of bed and walk some, with longer walks around the hallways every day. The more active a person is, the sooner he or she will go home, so walking is crucial. Some patients will go to physical therapy. The first day after the operation, a patient won't walk very far. Maybe to a chair, but that's it. A patient recovering well, however, will soon increase their distance walked along the hallways. Unless the patient has a high risk of falling, he or she can walk at will around the halls of the cardiac floor and enjoy the various window views.

The diet will be a cardiac one, and breakfast is remarkably bland, but you can basically have all you want to eat. (I recommend fruit and toast; avoid the eggs and potatoes.) Generally, it's no salt and no real butter. Patients typically have lost some weight, so if one isn't overweight, one can generally eat whatever they want within these parameters. I found the milkshakes were good, as were the sandwiches.

People will keep a close eye on each survivor of this operation. It isn't unusual to have irregular heartbeats for a day, as the heart doesn't like being touched. That's why patients wear a wireless heart monitor for their entire stay in the hospital. Nurse practitioners, patient care assistants, R.N.s, and assorted personnel – especially the cardiologist and the surgeon – will all be along to see how things are going. Patients who have had this operation will have a bandage vertically along the big sternum incision, and lots of tubes and wires hanging out, but this won't be a bother.

If one is on an IV, he or she can walk by rolling the portable IV stand. Patients don't get to shower due to the heart monitor, but can wash up with a washcloth. Patients can sit up in a chair and read (bring plenty of reading material) and talk on the phone. One should avoid a lot of family stress and try to be at peace. The chaplain's people will come by, and if one is Catholic, a lay minister will offer communion daily.

There is plenty of statistical evidence that people with any religious beliefs who pray or meditate recover faster than people who don't do so, and do better during the operation. Interpret that as you will, but the evidence is quite clear. Prayer, being at peace, meditation – whatever you call it – *speeds one's recovery*. Having a positive attitude, an attitude of "I have places to go and things to do," helps also. Put another way, being depressed about the operation after having survived it *isn't* helpful. A positive attitude and looking forward to being busy and doing things, is best.

Chapter 11: Going Home

The average person, whoever that is, leaves the hospital sometime within five to seven days after the operation. Patients are evaluated by physical therapy and social services personnel to see if the patient can function well in a home environment. Can the patients get up steps? Is someone home to cook meals? What level of post-hospital care will the patient need?

The doctor or nurse practitioner will decide when it's time to send the patient home. This could be a relatively surprising and short-notice decision. Really, the patient has been evaluated all along. Someone seeing the patient strolling around the hallways and enjoying the fine hospital meals and TV, especially on a weekday, is going to decide to review the chart with an eye to sending that patient home and making the bed available for another patient in need.

There is no point in *asking* to go home. Cardiac patients go when people decide they can go. My operation was on a Wednesday and I went home the following Monday evening at 6 p.m. It took three hours to finish the paperwork, get medicine at the hospital's pharmacy, and learn about post-hospital care.

In my case, the price of going home was to learn to give myself blood thinner shots in my stomach twice a day, for a week. If I couldn't deal with this emotionally, then I couldn't go home. I learned to do it under the instruction of a nurse. There was a lot of motivation to learn to stick a needle in my stomach if doing so meant I could go home and sleep all night.

Some younger people go home relatively easily. Other, often older people, head to a rehab center for a few weeks, then home. Each person's situation is unique, but in the best scenario, one goes home and back to where one feels comfortable and can sleep all night without being woken for blood pressure readings, etc.

No matter how well one feels in the hospital room, he or she will find that going home taxes one's endurance in getting from the hospital room into a car, and then getting into one's home. Some patients who head for a rehab center before going home need more time to find their strength, while others doing well go right on home, especially if they have someone there to help them. Patients typically have a visiting nurse stop by a couple times a week to check on them (provided insurance will cover these visits), but once at home with one's discharge instructions and medicines, the person is basically on their own. Recovery and getting back to work and other activities is up to each individual.

The doctors may call to see how the patient is doing, but recovery and getting on with life is the business of the patient. Unless there are complications, the patient is finished with the surgeon but will see the cardiologist the rest of their life. Some patients report feeling depressed, some hate the long scar down their sternum, and others worry about sudden valve failure all the time. Getting on with life is the job of the *patient* – it's not the family's job, nor the doctor's. Each person is very much on their own after the hospital stay, despite the follow-up visits. It's *your* life, so get on with it. Get out and be active.

The doctors and nurse practitioners will recommend walking, both while in the hospital and after discharge. One of my roommates while I was in the hospital not only never walked, but ate bad snacks all day and evenings, which his wife brought to the hospital. All day long, I could hear the two of them in the candy and potato chip bags. I suspect he had a brief life after going home.

Sometimes walking can be done at the hospital cardiac exercise center, which is a modern and reassuring place staffed by nurses that cost millions of dollars to build (often named after someone presumably important). Because it's full of heart patients, however, walking with another group or alone at the mall after discharge – surrounded by happy young shoppers – may be more reassuring than being surrounded by people with bad hearts. One won't be able to lift more than five pounds. There's no running or other fast movements, so as not to bounce that sewn-together sternum. No sitting in a bathtub, either, as this could cause infection. One gets showers and sex (hopefully), along with healthy food, walking, and sleeping.

Patients won't be allowed to drive for four weeks. An accident could crack apart the sternum, and potholes and bounces will hurt a lot, let alone having the energy to drive a car. Someone will have to drive the patient to early follow-up appointments, so take the heart pillow and hug it tightly while being driven. A bounce is going to hurt. Don't sneeze, either, as that will hurt even more. It's almost a *screaming* hurt, so stifle sneezes. The doctor should be consulted before driving, but most patients know when they can drive again. It'll be a few weeks.

Walking should be done when the patient feels the most energy, because the first few walks are going to tire the patient considerably. Walking even a block is a tough task when one is first home, as is walking up a flight of stairs. There is a temptation to not bother with the walks and just sit at home or, even *worse*, stay in bed all day. But walking is the number one way to a fast recovery, so one should gradually increase the distance and frequency of their walks. Combined with a cardiac diet and plenty of sleep, one may recover faster than expected. Sitting on the couch all day is *not* likely to promote a fast recovery, so get up and go outdoors. *Move around.* Do something during the day besides sleeping and sitting.

Chapter 12: Costs

Heart valve replacement is a major operation, with costs for the operation itself, hospital stay, doctors, consultations, and drugs somewhere in the plus-$250,000 range when I had it done back in 2009. Unless you have good insurance and drug coverage, this event could turn into a financial disaster. Some post-operative drugs require additional evaluation and testing, such as optical and pulmonary tests, due to side effects. Survivors of this operation will have numerous pills to take for the rest of their life for blood thinning, heart rhythm, blood pressure, cholesterol, etc., so hope for good drug insurance because the cost of drugs is going to add up in a hurry.

People who survive this operation will be required to take antibiotics an hour before *any* dental procedure to prevent an infection from getting into the heart valve area. Good gum health is related to good *heart* health, so heart patients should pay regular attention to their dental health. Antibiotics will need to be taken before dental procedures including routine teeth cleaning, gum work, and drilling.

Unfortunately, other medical concerns as a result of this operation will add even more to one's drug costs. One series of blood thinner shots I took at home cost $600 for 14 syringes (I had to give the injection myself, into my stomach area). Another drug was $100 for 30 pills *after* my insurance had paid. So be prepared. Good insurance and good drug insurance is crucial for preventing financial hardship, up to and including bankruptcy.

Chapter 13: Depression

A number of patients who go through this operation demonstrate symptoms of depression at various times afterwards. For some patients, the feelings of depression are often brought on by missing work for four to eight weeks, with much of the time spent sitting home alone, recuperating. Younger patients soon find, after returning home, that home life is going on very well without them because while they were in the hospital, the family learned to accomplish things without them. Suddenly, it doesn't seem to matter anymore what time the patient gets up in the morning, and in fact, oftentimes the family is better off without the patient being in the way while everyone is rushing to get ready for school and work. Old patients may discover their life partner is getting along just fine with no help from them, either.

This feeling of being *unessential* to the family carrying on can be troublesome to the patient – like a window to the future when the family really will go on without them. It's another thing not to think about.

Some patients fall into the trap of feeling that since the day is going to be spent sitting anyway, after doing their mandatory walking, there's little purpose in getting up at all. This is *not* a good outlook on life. People, even while at home, need to be engaging in hobbies, looking forward to future events, and talking to friends. Spending the day going for a walk, then sitting doing nothing except watching TV will likely lead to boredom and eventual distress.

In some measure, the patient's depression may be related to additional health problems separate from the operation. In addition, some people are bothered by the sight of the long sternum scar. It'll eventually fade, but it's noticeable for a while. Some are bothered by the pain in the sternum, but it will also fade. On rainy days, months later, the sternum is likely to ache, while on warm, sunny days, there will be no pain at all. Others are bothered by the constant checking of blood thinner levels, the concern about infections getting into the heart, or the endless cardiology appointments and monitoring. One rarely lives a carefree life after such an operation. Some people replay the hospital stay in their mind, over and over, instead of going out and living. One's point of view should be focused on living, not dwelling on the hospital stay, as this may encourage feelings of loneliness and isolation. The best course of action is to stay busy and sleep well at night.

Furthermore, from the patient's perspective, no longer being the center of the family's attention may reduce the importance of the operation, and themselves as a person, which can also lead to depression. There's a recognition of goals that won't be attained, that life is indeed brief and always terminal. This affects some patients seriously enough that they need medication for depression.

Activities and friends are good steps to avoiding depression. If, however, one *does* feel depressed, a consultation with a physician is clearly in order and should not be delayed.

I remember the night I left the hospital, sitting in my civilian clothing rather than a hospital gown in a hallway chair, holding a large fish balloon my son had given me while the housekeeping staff cleaned my room for the next heart patient. It was as if I'd never been there at all. My charts were gone, little packets of saved cracker snacks thrown away, my books packed up in my travel bag. I watched the nurses leaving together for a night out, smiling and happy to be off work, people going about their jobs while I sat in the hallway, waiting for my ride to come. People no longer checked on me, and no cheery comments came my way, such as "How are you doing today?" or "Feel better!" I was no longer on anyone's radar screen – there but not really *there* – because I'd been discharged. I was officially *gone*, just a person sitting in the hallway now, holding a balloon and wearing a black parka, waiting to go home. It was rather a letdown.

When a patient leaves the hospital after a big operation, they're likely to miss the attention, the safety, and the total experience of being a patient and being cared for. *Get over it*. If you're going home – and not to the funeral home – you should be smiling on your way out.

You lived through it.

Chapter 14: Does Life Change for the Better Afterwards?

People come to me and say, "You survived having your heart stopped while the doctors cut a piece out of your heart. Did your life change? Are you more spiritual now? Do you pray more, do you thank God, are your relationships better? Do you read the Bible daily as you did before the operation?" The simple answer is "No" to every question.

Don't assume one's life will suddenly change for the better. While people *can* change their lives, most go back to being what they were before the operation. There is rarely an epiphany about one's life after this operation that *changes* one's life. One may have prayed before the operation and read the Bible, but if one wasn't very religious before the operation, one probably won't be more so afterwards. One might use less salt and eat a little better, but overall, one's spouse and kids and friends will not love the patient any more than they did before the operation. A patient might go to church more, might think a little more about being good, and may even, in fact, be *nicer* to people and act better. Overall, though, it's unlikely one's personality will be drastically transformed.

If anything, there's a recognition that one's life expectancy may be somewhat more tenuous now. If the replacement valve fails, there probably isn't time to save the patient. That's a fact one *also* doesn't want to think about. It helps to keep busy and recognize that one may enjoy an experience that, without the operation, one wouldn't have survived to have. These experiences seem to make the operation worthwhile.

For me, after the operation, I went to see Montreal and listen to French. That was nice. My son and I went out in the rowboat one night and looked at the full moon. *That* was nice. I rode behind my son on a scale railroad at night with him running the locomotive in the dark, with the whistle sounding and the headlight shining on the rails. Mostly, I saw his blue jean jacket while he was sitting in front of me. That scene has been memorized. That night on the train with him was *more* than nice. The whole operation was worth living to experience that hour with my son. Perhaps you, as a survivor, will find some similar moments to cherish after your operation. If so, then it was worth doing.

I asked my son, assuming I won't still be alive to meet my grandkids in 10 years, if he'd tell them about me. He assured me he would. So, it's comforting to know that the things I did with *my* son, who was 10 at the time, will live on in the stories he tells *his* children. These sorts of reclamations of the future give patients hope that the operation was, indeed, *worth* it.

Chapter 15: Remembering

A lot of people took care of me after the operation. People I'll never see again. The stories they told of how they came to work at the hospital were remarkable, and a very valuable part of this whole experience.

There was the patient care assistant who was the only one of eight children who had a professional job. His mother had come to the US from West Africa to make a new life, and he had succeeded in life because of her. A nurse I talked to at 3 a.m. had come here from the Philippines for a better life, and she had over 20 years of experience. Another nurse told me a story of his mother who could never accept the death of her mother, and wasted her life pining for her. These stories are best heard between 2 and 4 a.m., when the floor is quiet, but you'll be awake while the nurses are tending to you.

You'll often be awake between 2 and 4 a.m., and 11 p.m. and 7 a.m., and just about every two hours or so, so sleep when you can. Healthcare professionals, in general, aren't shy about waking patients up when they need to talk or tend to them. As a result, one's sleep is always interrupted. Most doctors come through between 7 and 9 a.m., and they'll wake patients up, too. Don't expect to ever get a full night's sleep in the hospital. When one is ready for that, one goes home.

One nurse, while changing my sternum bandage, told me about her home in the South Pacific. I spent most of the story screaming and digging my nails into her leg as she removed and replaced the original bandage, but I also listened to her story as well as I could, under the circumstances.

That long sternum bandage has to come off and be changed, and this procedure is going to hurt. It's going to hurt a *lot*. But once the new bandage is on, the pain is gone. It only hurts while the nurse removes it, and only the first time. The nurses also wiped down the big incision with antiseptic several times a day. Infection in that incision is bad news and something everyone is very careful about. The last thing a patient wants, besides heart failure, is to get an infection that can go to the heart. Thus, the nursing staff is very careful around heart patients, especially ones with a long chest incision down the sternum.

Perhaps you'll spend time looking out the window and thinking about your life – what it was and what it will be. These thoughts often happen in the afternoon, when the sun is setting and the patient is waiting for dinner to arrive. What one's life was *before* the operation is in the past, and not likely to return. Former girlfriends and boyfriends don't suddenly reappear to relive and change the past. In all likelihood, what you have after the operation is what you're going to have in life.

A person will carry that long scar for a while. It'll fade eventually, but maybe not from one's mind. Perhaps you'll avoid going to the pool and beach shirtless, perhaps not. I never took my shirt off again at a pool, beach, or lake. Perhaps you'll be braver about that scar than I was. I could never stand the sight of it.

People ask if a survivor of this operation will be willing to scrap an unhappy life and start over for the sake of a better one. This willingness to completely change one's life and pour new people into it may largely depend on the age of the patient. If one is 80, there's probably no starting over. If one is 40...*maybe*. As with many things, tt depends upon the cost versus the expected improvement. Only the patient can decide. There's plenty of evidence that an unhappy, lonely life leads to heart trouble. That's something to consider when one is 35, not 80.

Research also shows that having friends and being happy, along with religion and spirituality, marriage, hobbies, and some steady values all contribute to a longer life after the operation. The best advice is to do as you wish, as being unhappy and miserable aren't productive, nor good for longevity. People either accept you or they don't, and nothing much you do will change their opinion of you, so carry on as you wish.

There's one sure thing to remember: being lonely in life is *not* good. Whether your friends are human, or you have a pet or spiritual friend, friendship is good for longevity. A happy marriage adds years to one's life too, especially for men.

On the day I went home, my cardiologist stopped in to say goodbye. I remember the day well. Cold, sunny, he came popping in suddenly at 2 p.m., bright and cheerful, and sat by the window with its fine view of a red brick wall. Tall, thin, young, he sat and looked at me. He was the same doctor who took the medical history when I was admitted through the ER, and the same doctor I still have. He came by as I was doing the final paperwork for leaving, which was a nice surprise. He said he wanted to get my thoughts on walking through the dark curtain and coming out alive.

I told him it was nice to be alive, and that I was somehow different, yet putting a finger on *how* I was different was difficult. I'd gained years of life by taking a risk that was best not thought about. I seemed more awake than before the operation, more aware, able to make connections more rapidly, and to think faster. He hadn't experienced the operation as I had, yet he certainly had seen a fair share of patients who had. In this regard, he was fascinated with people who survived and went on living, and curious to see how their lives turned out. When I saw him again for a checkup, I told him I'd been shoveling snow the day before. He smiled and wrote it down on the chart.

I guess the big effect of walking through the dark curtain is I can now shovel snow for hours and not feel tired. The winter of 2008-2009 in the Northeast was certainly a doozy. Snowstorm after snowstorm, with cold, bitter, icy weather all around.

I have no symptoms on the coldest and snowiest days now. That was a great improvement.

What Are Your Life Goals? Make a List!

Chapter 16: Later

There is one sure thing about this operation. If one survives, one is cured for as long as the valve lasts. While tissue valves need to be replaced eventually, an artificial valve may well outlast the patient. I was left with no symptoms after the operation. Today, years later, I can shovel snow for hours, walk in cold air, walk in hot air, exercise, run, and live an active life. It's as if I have the heart of a 25-year-old. It's amazing what raising the EF from 40 percent to 70 percent can do.

In 2009 in the Northeast, there were numerous big snowstorms. After the operation, I could shovel snow for hours with no symptoms at all. I can swing an ax again, split firewood, shovel gravel, row boats, and handle a chainsaw again. I can pick up four-foot long, 12-inch diameter logs. I can cut the grass. I can fight with an epee again. It was as if every month the heart became stronger, and in fact, my blood pressure steadily rose for the first four months after the operation – a testament to my heart's increasing ability to move blood.

There are two drawbacks. The first is the required medications. One will be on medication for the rest of their life. Blood thinners, Aspirin, blood pressure drugs, cholesterol-reducing drugs, and heart rhythm drugs are daily requirements for many people. *Any* procedure that might involve bleeding must be coordinated through the cardiologist. Future artery trouble or trouble with the artificial valve may require risky surgery, because to operate, the blood thinner that keeps the valve safely operating might have to be stopped. Stopping the blood thinner could mean serious trouble, and *fast*. A friend of mine had a general practitioner stop his Plavix for a mole removal, and he was dead in three days. The cardiologist was never consulted. It was a fatal medical error, and the general practitioner was sued by the widow.

The second drawback is that you *know* what's in your heart. An artificial piece of something is keeping your heart beating. Thinking about this is likely to make you nervous. The only solution is to keep busy, enjoy life, and try not to think about it.

These aspects aside, the operation does cure the problem, thus allowing great improvement in the quality and length of one's life. One may find the blood thinner checks become monthly, and the cardiologist visits go out to six months, with annual bloodwork and an annual echocardiogram.

For those who are afraid the valve will fail suddenly, counseling, getting in a positive frame of mind, being optimistic and hopeful, religious guidance, and talking with people who have survived the operation may help alleviate those fears. The operation is a scary procedure with weeks of recovery time, but the operation may well be the only reliable and generally successful cure. Unless one has mitigating factors, it's worth the risk to gain additional years in good health. I wish I'd done it as soon as I was diagnosed.

The operation turned my clock back by at least 20 years. So, *go*. Walk through the dark curtain with faith.

You'll be glad you took the chance.

Epilogue

The medical professionals who care for you see hundreds of the same cases every year, and answer the same questions over and over.

Some patients die. Some live. For everything there is a season. There's a time to die, and a time *not* to die.

If these professionals are curt with you or seem rushed, perhaps they've built good emotional firewalls for their own emotional survival. Just be glad they know their job well, which is to save your life. They may not have time to be chatty with you.

Be thankful they are there when you need them.

About the Author

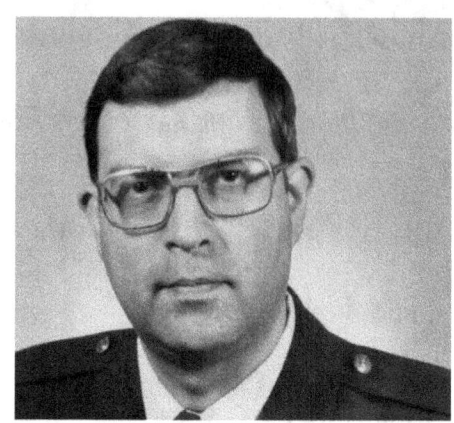

Dr. John Stibravy is a retired college professor and writer who lives in northern New Jersey. He coached the sport of fencing for many years. He had his first child, a son, at 50 years of age. His father lived to 96, and his grandmother lived to see 103. As of May 2022, he has survived his operation for more than 13 years.

He's the author of *I Was DEAD! Cardiac Arrest and My Journey Back to the Living*; *The Last Pretty Lake in New Jersey: Cedar Lake*; *Cardiac Arrest: Facts for Every American*; *World War I (56th Engineers) and Great Depression Letters of Ralph W. Green*; and *Dayton Steam: 1983 – 1992.*

About the Editor

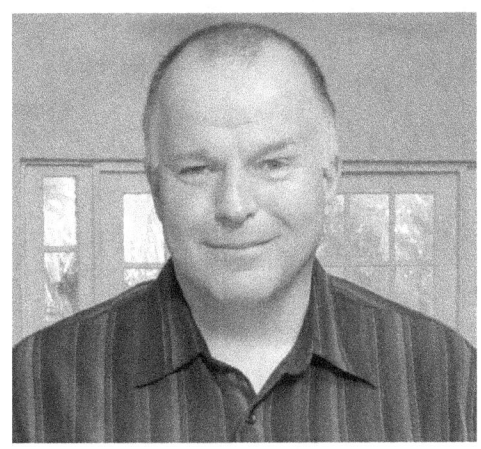

Tony Smith is a communication professor at St. Petersburg College in Florida. In April 2012, he was recognized as the third-highest rated professor in America on RateMyProfessors.com, and included in *The Best 300 Professors in America*, published by The Princeton Review.

He's the author of *Finish Your Damn Speech!* and *Strength on Wheels: What My '96 Cavalier Taught Me About Life* (available at Amazon). He's the narrator of this book and *Finish Your Damn Speech!* (available at Amazon, Audible, and iTunes).

He lives in Dunedin, Florida, and enjoys music, movies, hiking, photography, and playing basketball.